This digital edition published 2015.

Typesetting by Ian Ink

This book is not meant to replace any medical or professional advice delivered to you, or to counter or cure any pre-existing health condition.

This document is geared towards providing exact and reliable information in regards to the topic and issue covered. The publication is sold with the idea that the publisher is not required to render accounting, officially permitted, or otherwise, qualified services. If advice is necessary, legal or professional, a practiced individual in the profession should be ordered.

- From a Declaration of Principles which was accepted and approved equally by a Committee of the American Bar Association and a Committee of Publishers and Associations.

The information provided herein is stated to be truthful and consistent, in that any liability, in terms of inattention or otherwise, by any usage or abuse of any policies, processes, or directions contained within is the solitary and utter responsibility of the recipient reader. Under no circumstances will any legal responsibility or blame be held against the publisher for any reparation, damages, or monetary loss due to the information herein, either directly or indirectly.

Respective authors own all copyrights not held by the publisher.

The information herein is offered for informational purposes solely, and is universal as so. The presentation of the information is without contract or any type of guarantee assurance.

The trademarks that are used are without any consent, and the publication of the trademark is without permission or backing by the trademark owner. All trademarks and brands within this book are for clarifying purposes only and are the owned by the owners themselves, not affiliated with this document.

CONTENTS

Lean Vegan Exercise Routines

Introduction

First of all, let me say thank you for purchasing this book, and congratulate you on taking the very first step towards a healthier, fitter you! You will find in these pages that I have sought to formulate an easy guide to the Vegan Work-Out and lifestyle; one which can be started by anyone no matter their previous experience with dieting or exercise regimes.

Through the next few chapters I will present to you recipes, as well as exercise routines, hints and tricks, and some of the most successful strategies that I have employed for my own health.

Thanks again, and I hope that this book benefits you!

Veganism Explained

You may be already aware of what a vegan diet is, or you may have only ever heard about it in passing. No matter, this book will guide you through what veganism is, and also how it can benefit your body and mind.

Veganism is the dietary choice of trying not to knowingly ingest any animal products whatsoever; so, that means no meat, no fish, no dairy or milk, and no eggs or poultry products! Veganism is also a lifestyle choice as well as a dietary one, and so many vegans also choose to extend their prohibition to their shopping habits: only choosing clothes made from cotton and plant fibres, and not using any pharmaceutical or cosmetic items that have been tested on animals or use animal derivatives.

As I am sure that you can see immediately; the implications of a 100% vegan lifestyle and diet would be pretty vast, even just for one person!

This book will look at the vegan diet in particular, and will not focus on the vegan lifestyle. However it is worth noting that diet and lifestyle are very closely linked, and many people such as professional athletes, upon choosing this healthier option, also decide to adopt more humane ethical and non-animal practices throughout their life.

Don't Panic!

Obviously, you have come this far because you have an interest in the vegan diet – but still, you may feel a little overwhelmed by the change required in your diet. In many ways it is more difficult for those following a vegetarian diet to change to a vegan diet than for a 'general meat-eater' as the veggie diet relies very heavily on dairy products.

Well, let me encourage you not to panic. We're going to take this in small steps, it is perfectly okay to gradually become vegan, one meal at a time. I actually support a system of meal substitution rather than outright complete dietary overhaul, although you may differ. The final word of advice I would like to give is that, rather than when I started out as a vegan some ten years ago – there is now actually a large amount of vegan products available, as well as vegan-friendly labelling employed by many companies. The number of meat and dairy alternatives have sky-rocketed (for example: an alternative to milk used to be only soya or rice milk. Now there's hemp, almond, and hazelnut among others)!

Health Benefits of a Vegan Diet

To begin with, let us start by reviewing a few facts about an animal diet, which you may not already be aware of:

1. The average American has up to 5 pounds of undigested red meat in their gut at any time.
2. The human digestive system cannot cope with this high amount of meat intake, and the meat actually starts to decay inside the human body, releasing high amounts of nitrogen and other nasty chemical enzymes before it leaves our body.
3. Almost all animal red-meats suffer from being given animal growth hormones to 'bulk them up' for the supermarkets, or alternatively steroids and antibiotics to stave off the diseases of living in close quarters. These are passed on in their meat to the human, whose immune system becomes compromised, and under pressure.
4. Because plant-based sources of nutrition are less complex than animal based sources, they are more easily digested by the human body, allowing our body access to the essential minerals, nutrients, and enzymes contained within. This notion is called bioavailability of nutrients.
5. The modern (Western) diet is heavily concerned with producing and eating animal products, as well as high calorie sugar and carbohydrate products. This endless press of snacks and take-away foods are almost designed to keep us eating, and not exercising. Breaking free of this habit is therefore essential for a healthy lifestyle!

6. A plant-based diet is lighter on the body, leaving you feeling more refreshed, agile, and non-lethargic!
7. A plant-based diet, thanks to all of the benefits outlined above, places less strain on our own human growth hormones, as well as our immune and endocrine systems, resulting in a more stable sleep cycle, a healthier immune system, and faster recovery rate when we exercise.

What's So Bad About Dairy, Anyway?

One of the reasons why many professional athletes choose to move beyond dairy is because of the physical affects that dairy products have on the body. You may have heard of the old adage that dairy products promotes colds or weight issues (due to their high fat content) but, if we look further there is also an alarming correlation between dairy and all sorts of very serious health concerns.

Let us now turn to give a very brief overview of why dairy can be bad for the health-conscious individual.

1. Although dairy is often high in protein, it is also very high in fats. These fats are hard to metabolize, and means that your body has to fight off a weight increase rather than concentrate on a muscle increase!
2. Dairy is, essentially, baby-food. It is high in all of minerals and trace elements that pass through a cow, sheep, and goat's udders. Unfortunately, in today's day and age of modern industrial farming, that means that these livestock also pass on animal growth hormones, cattle steroids, as well

as heavy metals from their diets. In baby calves these promote fattier tissue, excellent for beef cattle, but terrible for human cells.

3. Milk proteins from other animal species are actually far larger than the ones produced through human pregnancy (just think of the structure difference between cows and humans). In digesting them, the human digestive tract actually inflames (leading to the bloated, queasy feeling you might have after too much chocolate or milk deserts). Our own cell receptors often rupture when trying to digest these larger protein molecules, putting a strain on our immune system.

4. Milk products do not deliver high-available protein (for the above reason) and so, many professional athletes decide to eat protein sources which are more closely aligned to our own bodies natural abilities: nuts and seeds!

Vegan Shopping

Despite the ease of living a vegan lifestyle in today's day and age, and despite the many alternatives to an animal-based diet there are – it can sometimes be a challenge to ensure that you have access to the non-animal food. That is why it is important, at the start of your journey, to consider a few points.

Tip: Before you start, take a search through your local, usual shopping outlet for non-animal products. Usually there will be a section entitled 'meat-free' or 'animal-friendly' or similar. Also, consider looking at the cheaper, own-brand foods, as these are often made without recourse to animal products!

Tip: Start your diet and work out lifestyle by preparing a few of the delicious snacks and light bites outlined in the recipe section (Part 2!). If you prepare them now, that means that if you are caught out, not knowing where to find a particular item or foodstuff, then you will have food prepared to keep you going!

Tip: I cannot impress on you the importance of visiting your local fruit and vegetable market (particularly if it is also organic) as well as your local health/whole food establishment. Usually these purveyors are a wealth of local and nutritional information, and their support in your plant-based diet will become invaluable. You never know – they might also know of a good running club or gym class as well!

Step 1

- *Find out where the meat-free aisles and sections are in your usual shopping haunts.*
- *Find out where your local health and whole food stores are, as well as veg markets.*

PART 1: The Vegan Work-Out Diet Explained

The Vegan Work-Out diet works on a very simple principle: some proteins and nutrients are easier to absorb by your body than others. Added to this, is the idea that if we seek to minimize the pressure that we put on our digestion, and accompany that with a more natural style of exercising, then we will be giving our body its maximum health potential.

This Work-Out Diet is not about intensive exercises designed to just do one thing for your body such as bulking up, getting 'cut' (muscle definition). This exercise plan and diet is about the wholeness of your bodies systems, not just one part of your physical health over another.

This Work-Out diet is not also about extreme dietary requirements and strictures: counting such and such calories, or only eating this type of food on day 3 or day seven, or perhaps of starving your body into submission. No, no, *no!*

The Lean Vegan Work-Out Diet is about providing the best environment for your body, both internally and externally. You may have heard of the idea of Holism, which is one which has a lot of resonance for us in this book. Holism means looking at the system as a whole, and trying to achieve balance through all of it. For example, if you wish to become fitter, you don't *just* go running three times a week, but ignore your diet or continue to eat doughnuts and cake every night!

In the same way, this book seeks to address your body as a *whole* unit. We will try to give your body exactly what it needs, and nothing that it doesn't need, as well as giving it the sorts of exercises that it evolved to perform.

One of the ideas that I think makes sense is that humans have never been fitter than when we lived a Palaeolithic lifestyle. We would eat an overwhelmingly plant-based diet, and we would be constantly active. But we wouldn't over-burden our bodies with just one type of exercise (like power lifting, or marathon runners). Instead, we would ask our bodies to perform a range of movements and exercises, and all of these exercises would increase our *whole* general health.

***Tip:** It is actually well known that one health exercise, to the detriment of a well-rounded health regime can be severely damaging Many power-lifters suffer from heart complaints in later life, as their heart struggles with that much mass to move around!*

To that end, the Lean Vegan Work-Out Diet will seek to provide you with easy, light foods that are light on your stomach, enabling you to move, and enabling your body to take advantage of their nutrients. This is a vitally important point: that much of modern, processed food is actually very hard to digest, and our body cannot unlock their nutrients in any meaningful way, leading us to become malnourished!

Going back to our earlier idea of the Palaeolithic diet, and giving our body what it needs – we have to remember that our Palaeolithic ancestors ate entirely natural foods – not processed foods of any kind. Our digestion hasn't changed that much, and the high-processed foods such as sugars, syrups, and ready-meals are hard to break down and yield less benefit than a directly plant-based diet.

Tip: Eat natural where you can, and try to eat organic and whole food wherever possible. Most processed foods will be refined, meaning that they are heavy in one particular nutrient, sugar, or fat. Your body actually needs a whole variety of nutrients and minerals to digest at the same time, as each enzyme helps to unlock others.

Again, ask your local Health/Whole food store about this.

Meal Diary

So, you want to be lean, mean and fit, right? You want the body of your dreams? You want to be as healthy as those ancestors that walked across the Sahara, sailed across the pacific, climbed the Alps – all without modern technology?

Good! To start with, you are going to have to work out what you are eating currently, in order to know how to change it!

We've all had that moment when we start a new project or health routine, but after a week or a month the enthusiasm fails, and we suddenly realize that we have given up without even knowing why! That is why it is important, with such a big change as going vegan, to take things slowly and to prepare. Our first step will be what we call the Meal Diary.

The Meal Diary is a tool for you to work out what you are eating currently (where healthy or ill), as well as to chart your progress with your Lean Vegan Work Out Diet. You will find that this simple little exercise will manage to provide you almost invaluable information when followed assiduously, such as;

- *When do you eat 'comfort food'? Is there a particular time of the day, or time in the week?*
- *Why do you eat comfort food?*
- *When is your day very busy, and it is easier to get snacks or readymade meals than to make or prepare your own?*
- *What meals during the week could you exchange and substitute for other, healthier options?*
- *When does your body start getting tired, and need an energy boost throughout the day?*

To start with, simply use a normal pocket day-planner or you could use a wall-planner calendar. It is important there is enough space each day to report on every food and drink that passes your lips!

Keep a running total or your meals snacks, and drinks. Note everything from cups of coffee to main meals, take-away sandwiches to chocolate bars. You can go into detail and also account their calories, or you could just list it such as coffee's: 3, sandwich: 1, salad: 1 and so on.

Just by keeping a record of what you have eaten on each day will give you a good picture of your eating habits. You may be surprised at what and when you do and do not eat. Many of us in the modern world exist on a sort of 'starve & graze' system, where we are too busy for long periods of the day to prepare a meal when our body needs it, but when we have our work breaks we will fill up on snacks, or eat mindlessly through the next few hours. It is these mental habits that we will be addressing with the Lean Vegan Diet and Work Out as much as our choice of food.

Tip: If you also note down the time of each meal or beverage, and perhaps a note about the sort of day you are having, such as 'busy – full day at work' or 'worked late' or 'half day' then you will have an invaluable amount of information. You will see that your body starts to get tired at certain times, and that you usually answer that tiredness with this and that regular foodstuff or drink (coffee and snacks, for most of us!). By being fore-armed, you will also be forewarned, and simply by supplementing and substituting those snacks at that time of the day (making sure you have a tasty salad in your bag at eleven o'clock) you will save yourself a lot of heartache and calories!

The Diet Plan

The next step, after you have started a Meal Diary is to complete the Diet Plan. You will find that it is a sort of natural extension of the above, and the more time you spend on the Meal Diary, the more that it will naturally evolve into the Diet Plan of its own accord.

You will need; another wall-planner, calendar or notebook, (or just a few pieces of paper), and in this you will divide the space into the days of the week. In here you will list the meals that you will be substituting for your normal, non-diet meals.

This will also become your roadmap and a record of your experiment. As you progress with the Lean Vegan Diet, you will find that some meals might work better on some days (when you have more time to prepare them, for example) and that this diet plan fits almost perfectly with your Exercise Plan (Part 3)!

By the time that you are familiar with this book, we want you to have a record of what you *can* do to change your diet, and how you *have*. This will include the meals that you have exchanged and what you have eaten when, as well as the certain days when these or those exercises are preferable.

Tip: Use separate calendars and notebooks to start, but as you progress, put all of the information into a big diary journal, held especially just for your Lean Vegan Diet. In this book you will have details of your exercises, meals, as well as tips and notes on what you might do to enhance or avoid. Add recipes and notes on things that you might want to try!

Substitution & Being Prepared.

Are you ready to begin the Lean Vegan Diet? You have your Meal Diary and your Diet Plan ready? Great, then let's begin…

You have been faithfully recording your non-diet meals in your Meal Diary. Now, with your Diet Plan you are going to choose one meal *for every day of the week* and substitute it with one of the recipes outlined in Part 2. It could be a Breakfast, a Main Meal, a Snack or similar, but remember to vary it throughout the weak, so that you will experience the full range of benefits of the vegan diet.

In the next week of the Diet, you will add vegan meals to that Diet Plan, substituting more of your non-vegan meals with purely vegan ones, until your week is full of a purely Lean Vegan Diet recipes!

In this gradual way – even if you are already vegetarian or vegan, you will be allowing your body to adjust as well as to detox as you exercise. Instead of a sudden change in lifestyle and eating habits, you will slowly add more healthy and better foodstuffs along with more strenuous exercises, until after a month or two you won't even recognise the old you!

Tip: The key to substitution and the Diet Plan is being prepared, which, thankfully you are because of your Meal Diary. You will be able to see the times of the day when you get tired and reach for quick food, and also the days on which you usually have more time to cook a bigger meal. By choosing these crucial times, and thinking creatively about your diet, you will ensure that your normal day-to-day life is unaffected, just enhanced!

Step 2

- *Create a Meal Diary, over at least one week. Chart every non-diet food and drink that you eat.*
- *In week 2, create a Diet Plan in the same or separate journal/notebook/planner. Choose one Lean Vegan recipe solution for each day. This could be a breakfast, a main meal, or a snack or similar.*
- *Make sure that you have time to prepare the ingredients and get to the shops that you discovered in Step 1 (it is a good idea, at this early stage, to prepare a few of these meals in advance, to save you having to worry about it mid-week).*

PART 2: Vegan Recipes

Breakfasts

Pure Porridge

- ⅄ 1 cup of organic porridge oats
- ⅄ 2 cups of soya, hemp, or nut milk of your choice
- ⅄ A handful of dried currants to sweeten

One of the great things about soya, rice and hemp milk is that it naturally tastes a little sweeter than cow's milk, so it is easier to add to porridge and cereals without the need to add sugar or honey! Instant calorie buster!

Simply add your chosen milk alternative to a cup of porridge oats in a pan on the hob, heat through gently until the oats start to congeal and add your currents as you cook! Only takes 5-7 mins to prepare.

Forager's Muesli

- ⅄ 1/2 cup of wholefood, organic Muesli
- ⅄ 1 Apples, peeled and chopped.

- ⚘ Handful of currents and or dried fruit.

- ⚘ Handful of cashews or whatever mixed nuts that you have

- ⚘ 2 cups of soya, hemp, or nut milk of your choice

Simply put together as you would any normal cereal or muesli, but use your fresh fruit, dried berries and selection of nuts and seed to make it extra tasty and nutritious! Good to keep you going for the whole morning!

Drinks - Juices

Blue Apple-Juice

- 1 cup of Blueberries.
- 2 Apples, peeled and cored.

Juice all of the ingredient together and you're good to go! Put into fridge-freezer if you want a thicker, cold drink.

Apples 'n' Pears

- 2 pears (skinned and stalk removed).
- ½ peeled lemon.
- 3 cored and peeled apples.

Juice all of the ingredients together, and consume!

Sun-in-a-Jar!

- 1 Peach (without pits).
- 8 Strawberries.
- 1 Banana, peeled.
- ½ Mango, peeled.

Place everything in the juicer or blender, and blend!

Mango Zing.

- 1 Apple, cored but not peeled (cut in half, and remove the harder core).

- 1 Peeled Orange (it's going to be messy!)

- ½ Lemon, peeled.

- ½ teaspoon of cinnamon.

Juice everything together and serve with ice-cold water. Prepare your taste-buds to be zing'ing!

B – Healthy

- 1 tablespoon of fresh Parsley.

- 1 Cucumber.

- 2 Celery stalks.

- 2 Carrots.

- 1 handful of Spinach.

Put all together and drink as a 'green' juice. Add to your morning regime to help your immune-system throughout the day.

- 1 teaspoon of Wheat Grass

Sugar Nectar ('Bounce-Juice')

⅄ 2 Nectarines, pitted.

⅄ Peeled Guava.

Juice together and drink. Get ready to take on the world!

Drinks - Smoothies

Heal-All Smoothie

- ⚶ 1 Banana, peeled and chopped.
- ⚶ ½ cup of Raspberries.
- ⚶ 1 cup of oat or rice milk.

Blend the Banana and Raspberries together, and then juice with the oat or rice milk. To make this drink even more nutritious, consider adding small amounts of Wheatgrass!

Big-Berry Bonanza

- ⚶ 1 Banana, peeled and chopped.
- ⚶ 8-10 Strawberries.
- ⚶ ½ cup of Blueberries.
- ⚶ ½ cup of Raspberries.
- ⚶ 2 cups of oat or rice milk.

Blend everything together in a blender, and then put into fridge-freezer for a 2 minutes. Delicious and nourishing.

Cricketing Summer

- 10 Strawberries.

- 1-2 cups of Almond Milk.

- A few sprigs of mint, chopped.

Blend the fruit and milk all together, and mix. Add the mint after wards, on-top.

Light Meals - Soups & Stews

Borscht

- ⅄ 1 chopped Onion.

- ⅄ 2 Carrots, peeled and chopped.

- ⅄ 2 Potatoes, peeled and diced.

- ⅄ 6 Beets, peeled and chopped.

- ⅄ Large handful of Spinach (or Kale).

- ⅄ One small tray of fresh tomatoes (a tin of chopped at a pinch)!

- ⅄ 3 Tablespoons of fresh chopped Parsley.

- ⅄ 2 teaspoons of white or cider vinegar.

- ⅄ Pepper, Salt and Bay Leaves to flavor.

Lightly fry the beets in fresh oil for 2 minutes, place into a bowl and mix in the vinegar.

Lightly fry the onion at the bottom of a soup pot, when slightly golden-soft add the potatoes, carrots parsley and spinach and add stock water with seasoning (7-10 cups of warm water).

Simmer all the vegetables until cooked, (10-20 minutes), add the tomatoes and beets and 'cook-in' for a few more minutes. Garnish with vegan sour cream-cheese!

Black-Bean Soup

- 2 cups of Black Beans, rinsed (or 1 tin).

- 2-4 Garlic cloves, chopped and diced.

- 1 large Tomato.

- 1 chopped white Onion.

- Salt, Olive Oil, Veggie Stock, White or Cider Vinegar and Black Pepper to taste.

- 1 teaspoon-tablespoon of Cumin.

In one pot place the Black Beans into a soup pot of stock and bring to the boil and then gently simmer for 2 hours. Add salt.

Gently fry the garlic and onion in a pan with a light amount of oil, add the tomato and cumin. When fried off, add to the Black Bean mixture, add the vinegar and mix. Heat the broth through and reduce for another fifteen minutes.

Potato & Leek Heart-Warmer

- ⚔ 1 large Onion, chopped.

- ⚔ 1 chopped Leek.

- ⚔ 3 heaped tablespoons of vegetable margarine.

- ⚔ 3 medium Potatoes, peeled, chopped and cubed.

- ⚔ 2 cloves of Garlic, chopped and diced.

- ⚔ 3 cups of oat milk.

- ⚔ Paprika, Pepper, Salt and Parsley to flavor.

Gently fry the Onion, Leek and Garlic together (keep away from your eyes!) with the margarine.

When the mixture is soft add the oat milk, paprika, pepper and parsley and mix. Remember to use a soup pot! Add the potatoes and cook until potatoes are soft, 15-20 minutes.

When all ingredients are soft, serve!

Hot-Broth Soup!

- Vegetable noodles (soya or thin rice noodles).

- 2 handfuls of baby Spinach, washed.

- ¼ teaspoon Cayenne pepper.

- ¼ teaspoon fresh Ginger, grated, chopped and chopped again!

- ¼ teaspoon Black pepper.

- ¼ cup of rice, cider or Balsamic vinegar.

- 5-6 cups of vegetable stock.

- 2 tablespoons of raw, natural sugar.

In a large soup pot, add the stock water and bring to the boil, stir in the vinegar, pepper, ginger and Cayenne pepper and sugar. Reduce the heat and allow to simmer for 6-10 minutes. Add the spinach and your vegan noodles, simmer for a further 6 minutes.

Remove from the heat, allow the pot to stand for 4-5 minutes to cool and mix before serving.

Light Meals – Salads

Vegan Caesar Salad

- Handful of sliced Almonds
- 3 Cloves of Garlic
- ¼ lb of silken/light tofu
- 1 large lettuce
- Handfuls of whatever leafy greens you have (spinach, rocket)
- A few sprigs of mint, chopped.
- Fresh black pepper and sea salt to season
- 2 tablespoons of lemon juice

Chop and blend the almonds, then set aside. Chop the green salad leaves into an arrangement of your choice, and set aside.

Using a clean blender, combine the garlic, tofu, a heavy drizzle of virgin olive oil and lemon juice until a thick sauce has been created. If not combining, simply add a little more olive oil. Add pepper and salt to taste, and drizzle over your salad leaves!

Vegan Bean Salad

- 1 tin of edamame beans (or whatever you have in the cupboard)
- 1 small tin of black-eyes peas
- 3 teaspoons of; vinegar, sesame oil, and soy sauce,
- Black pepper and sea salt to taste.

Wash and rinse the tinned beans, and place in a pan of near-boiling water. Boil for no more than 5 mins, then drain and combine with the wet ingredients! Add pepper and salt to taste, or a drizzle of lemon juice. You can always add any roasted seeds such as sesames, cashews or sunflower seeds for texture and a smokier taste.

Vegan Roasted Salad

- 1 head of fennel, chopped into chunks
- 2 large shallots, peeled and chopped
- 1 Aubergine, chopped into chunks
- Green leafy veg of your choice
- A generous drizzle of olive oil, vinegar and nut oil

⅄ Pepper and salt to taste

Rub the fennel, shallots and Aubergine with a generous nut oil, then place on a roasting tray in the oven for 30-45 mins, at 200C/350F. They should crisp and start to brown, but remain juicy. Combine on a plate with your chosen green leafy veg, a generous drizzle of olive oil, vinegar, and nut oil.

Add pepper and salt to taste.

Main Meals

Simple Potato Curry

- 4 Large potatoes, peeled and cubed.
- 1 medium Chili pepper, chopped fine.
- Tomato paste (a good dollop).
- Handful of chopped Coriander (finely chopped).
- ½ teaspoon of Mustard seeds.
- 2-4 teaspoons of Cumin.
- 1-2 teaspoons of curry powder.
- Vegetable oil, lemon juice, and salt as needed.

Boil the potatoes in a separate pan until tender and then drain, and leave to one side.

Gently fry the Cumin, curry spaces, pepper and tomato in another pan for 1 minute, add Mustard seeds. Add the potatoes to the mixture, and gently stir all together, adding lemon juice and Coriander as needed for piquancy. Serve alone, as a side dish or with rice!

Long Mongo Daal

- 6 oz/180g whole Mung Beans, washed.

- 5-7 cloves of garlic, chopped and diced.

- 2 medium Onions, chopped.

- ¾ lb/340g of Tomatoes, chopped (or a tin)!

- ½ lb/225 g fresh Spinach leaves, washed and chopped.

- Olive oil, salt, lime juice to flavor.

- Fenugreek, Cumin to taste.

First, prepare the Mung Beans by washing and placing in a pot and bringing to the boil. Take off the heat and allow to stand for 1 hour. Bring the Beans to the boil once again and leave to simmer on a low heat for 1 hour.

Whilst you are on your second boil of the Mung Beans, place the onion, garlic and spices in a pan and saute with oil until soft and the spices are fried off. Add the tomatoes, stir together and fry for a further 5-6 minutes and add Spinach, salt and lime juice.

When the Spinach has begun to soften, add the Mung beans and bring to a simmer. Simmer for a further 5 minutes and until cooked. Allow to sit for 1-2 minutes to cool before serving!

Pasta Sauce

- 4 cloves of garlic, chopped finely.

- 1 large chopped Onion.

- 5 cups of chopped Tomatoes (fresh is preferable).

- Handful of diced olives (no stones).

- Handful of fresh Basil.

- Teaspoon of fresh Rosemary.

- Olive oil, salt and pepper, teaspoon of Balsamic Vinegar.

Heat the garlic, onions and oil together until soft, add the Rosemary, tomatoes and Basil; simmer for 15 minutes. At this point you can remove from the heat and puree if you want a thin consistency, or leave slightly lumpy!

Return to the heat and add the Olives and the Balsamic and simmer on a reduced heat for 10 more minutes.

Pour over cooked pasta! If you want to make an especially rich Bolognese, add chopped mushrooms when you are frying your Onions and garlic (with a little more oil to compensate), and maybe even some Vegan mince!

Veggie Enchiladas

- 1-2 Red Onions, chipped.

- 4 Garlic cloves, chopped fine.

- 8 teaspoons of whole wheat flour

- 1 cup assorted vegetables/tofu slices (anything chopped or cubed fairly small).

- 10+ Large corn tortillas (available from any supermarket).

- 1 Chili pepper, chopped and diced.

- 1 teaspoon Cumin.

- 1/s cup of Tamari.

- Water, salt and pepper as needed.

- Veggie cheddar cheese (shredded or grated).

Lightly fry the onion and garlic in oil, add chili, cumin, tamari and water. Be careful of spitting hot chili water or oil – stand well back if already hot. Gently shake in the flour evenly to the pot, stir and simmer. Allow 8 minutes for the sauce to thicken.

With your choice of leftovers, make sure all are cooked either by briskly frying, steaming or boiling for 5-7 minutes. Fill each prepared tortilla with the vegetables and roll together. Place with the overlapping seam 'down' on an oiled baking tray in the oven.

Spread your thickened sauce and the crumbled cheese over the filled tortillas, and bake in a preheated oven for 20 minutes, or until the cheese has melted and started to caramelize-brown.

Nut Loaf!

- ⚔ 3 parsnips, cooked and mashed
- ⚔ 2 small onions, chopped
- ⚔ 3 cloves of garlic, crushed
- ⚔ 8 oz. (200g) cashew nuts, ground
- ⚔ 8oz. (200g) mushrooms, finely sliced.
- ⚔ 1 tablespoon of cornflour
- ⚔ 1 small handful of chopped chives
- ⚔ A teaspoon of chopped thyme
- ⚔ 100ml veg stock, and a dollop of Yeast Extract.

To first prepare the parsnips, boil or steam until starting to go soft and set to one side. Fry the onions and garlic in a separate pan with oil, when cooked add to a bowl with the cashew nuts, cornflower and herbs.

Add the mashed parsnips, mixing everything together thoroughly.

Fry the mushrooms in the old Onion pan until soft and add to the mixture. Dissolve the yeast extract into the stock water (use warm water) and add to the mixture until thoroughly moist. Mix all of the ingredients together well.

Place the mixture into a prepared baking 'loaf

tin', already greased (this stops it sticking at the bottom). Fold over a piece of tin foil over the top, and bake for approximately 45 mins – 1 hour. Serve when taken out and has cooled down for 5 minutes.

Shepherdess' Pie

- 1 small Onion, chopped.

- 1 Leek, chopped.

- 1 large Carrots, peeled and chopped.

- 8-10, 2 pounds or 800g of Potatoes, skinned and chopped.

- 100g of Soya/Veggie Mince.

- 1 pint vegetable stock

Bring the washed and skinned potatoes to a boil in a large pan, and then lower the heat to simmer in the background.

Fry your Leek and Onion together, until they start to caramelize. Add Carrots and stock and simmer until carrots are starting to soften (5-10 minutes). Add the Veggie Mince, salt, pepper and any additional flavorings (2-3 Bay leaves?) and allow to simmer for a few more minutes, mixing the filling all together.

If you like a sharper taste, at this point you can add a tin of chopped tomatoes and some oregano!

Pour the mixture in an oven-proof dish and top with mashed potatoes. Place in over and ready to eat after baking for 30 minutes!

Vegan Risotto

- 1 tray/200g of Mushrooms, sliced.

- 1 medium Onion, chopped.

- 1 red Pepper (not a hot Pepper), chopped.

- 1/3 cup of Cauliflower florets, chopped fairly small.

- 100g of Brown, or Pot Rice

- I large handful of either sunflower seeds, or cashew nuts.

Fry the Onion off in a pan until starting to caramelize. When this happens, add in the mushrooms and pepper and saute together (adding extra oil where needed). Add the Cauliflower florets and cook through for a few more minutes. Pour in about half to a pint of stock water and add the rice. Leave to simmer for 25 minutes, or until the rice is cooked.

Reduce the mixture and add the nuts and seeds of your choice. Drain excess and serve with lashings of Soy sauce (Tamari, Black Bean or favorite).

Deserts & Snacks

Carrot Cake

- ⚕ 2 cups whole-wheat flour.

- ⚕ 1-2 cups natural brown sugar.

- ⚕ ⅓ cup of vegan margarine.

- ⚕ 4 cups grated carrot.

- ⚕ 1 teaspoon vanilla extract.

- ⚕ 1 teaspoon cinnamon.

- ⚕ A scattering of smashed/ground cardamom seeds.

- ⚕ ¼ teaspoon ground ginger (or use fresh, but very finely grated and chopped).

- ⚕ 2 teaspoon baking powder1 teaspoon baking soda.

- ⚕ ⅓ cup vegan cream cheese.

- ⚕ 2 ⅓ cups icing sugar.

- ⚕ 1 cup of fresh vegetable oil.

Mix all the dry ingredients together in a bowl (the flour, baking powder, bicarb and sugar). Add in the oil, your grated carrots and mix together thoroughly. It should have a 'gloopy' or stodgy texture.

Pour into a baking pan and cook in a preheated over for between 35-45 minutes, until the center is dry.

Whilst the cake is cooling, smoosh the icing sugar, margarine and cream cheese together until well mixed. Continue to mix, adding the vanilla essence as you do, until the texture is smooth and has little granular 'pockets' or bubbles.

Ladle, spoon r pipe the icing sugar onto the carrot cake, and crumble the ground cardamom on top as a 'garnish'.

Apple Roly-poly

- 2 medium-sized apples, sliced.
- 170g self-raising flour (wholemeal).
- 85g vegan margarine
- 1-2 large dollops of red jam, sprinkles of a natural raw cane sugar.

'Smoosh' the flour and margarine together between your fingers, mix with water to make a sweet dough and roll out into your desired shape.

Spread the sweet dough with the jam (forming a mortar paste), and layer the thinly sliced apples onto the mixture. Sprinkle the whole with with sugar and roll the shape, folding over and sealing the ends tight.

Place in an oven dish and bake until golden! Serve with custard, vegan cream or vegan ice cream!

Shortbread

- 100g white plain flour (organic preferable).
- 100g vegan margarine
- 50g raw cane sugar

Sieve the flour and sugar together into a bowl, knead together the margarine. When the shortbread is fully mixed, pack into a small, pre-greased baking tin.

Place at the bottom of your oven and cook for about 45-50 minutes, until golden color on top! Sprinkle the top with the raw cane sugar as soon as it comes out of the over, helping it to bond with the top!

Step 3

- *Replace 1 meal a day from your normal Meal Diary with one of the vegan recipes. Do this for a week.*
- *In week 2, try to replace two meals a day of your normal diet with a vegan recipe.*
- *By week 3, replace all three meals a day of your normal diet with the vegan recipes above!*
- *For week 4, start experimenting by finding your own vegan recipes, and trying out new vegan snacks to eat.*

PART 3: The Vegan Work-Out

Getting Started

Now that you have made a start with a vegan diet, you will find that you are actually generating a lot more energy, stamina, and interest in an active life. All of those heavy dairy products that naturally bloat the body, give you headaches and make you feel tired will be out of your system – leaving you feeling refreshed and lighter.

The key to any exercise routine is to start light, and to constantly challenge yourself. This can be a subtle point for someone new to exercising – but remember the axiom:

It's all about balance!

A healthy body gets fitter, stronger, faster, and more flexible in response to a constant, low-level stimulus. It does not get fit when overwhelmed with impossibly hard tasks – that way strains, tears, and sports injuries lie! For example, if you were not an experienced hiker, and yet you took to climbing a mountain very quickly, you would expect to get blisters or perhaps even a strained ankle. The same goes for exercise.

What we will be doing is introducing a light routine to your week, then, as your stamina grows, we will increase the load and strain of that routine gradually. Your body will adapt by trimming off the fat and becoming leaner in response to the exercise, utilizing all of that healthy bio-available nutrients that you have been feeding it with!

The Golden Formula

There are many websites and articles out there that will tell you the golden formula to getting fit is this or that set of exercises. I am about to let you in on a secret; in actual fact *no one knows* the golden formula that will work for *your* body. Or, to put it another way – only you do!

Tip: Learn to listen to your body. Listen to what areas ache, what areas feel tight. Pay especial attention to the morning after an exercise day. How tight are your muscles and tendons? Learn how strong you are. At first this can be a bit of a balancing act, but by approaching exercise with a little bit of caution – you should be fine!

However; a little bit of sports and nutritional science can help us in understanding the business of exercise...

Your body is an engine. It runs on the many different types of nutrient fuel that you feed it – primarily protein, some essential fats, and a whole lot of vitamins, minerals, and water. This fuel keeps your muscles healthy, your organs working properly. Your bodies' endocrine system also generates enzymes to regulate your hormones, immune system, metabolism and general health; which is directly affected by how active you are, and how healthy you eat.

Conclusion: Healthy food + Activity = leads to a healthier you!

Sometimes, however, we want to take this a little bit further and to actually lose weight and to counter any previous health ailments or bad habits. This is where the nutritional science and exercise comes in.

Your body uses the energy that is available, and, for most of us, it is quicker (but not easier) for our body to use sugars as a quick burst of energy. We either get this from sugary snacks, processed food, or our body makes the sugar from carbohydrates such as bread, pasta, wheat products. We use this energy as we need, but our body is also addicted to this process of 'releasing energy' – it is the very reason why many of us have a sweet tooth! We consume and release more energy than we need to, and our body has to metabolize that energy back into 'storage'.

The way that our body stores energy (sugar and carbs) is to metabolize it into fats, which is why, when we eat without burning the energy off, we get larger. Our body has gone into over-storage mode.

The above becomes a type of vicious cycle when we also add in the fact that it is easier for our body to get lots of sugary energy, but harder for our body to get the actual wholefood, complex nutrients and vitamins that it needs (why many of us take supplements every day as well). Your body asks for the types of building blocks it needs, and we fail to give it, so it slows down. Our metabolism starts to slow, making the burn-off rate of sugar to energy slower, and the conversion of sugar to fat easier. We get fatter, slower, and unhealthier.

One of the key things that we will be doing to counter this, is to raise our metabolic rate. Luckily, this is quite easy to do. Between 20 mins to 45 mins of a raised heart rate is usually enough to trigger our metabolic rate to raise, often producing a light sweat, and forces our body into 'use energy! Convert stored fat to energy!' (Or as we call it – losing weight).

Now, there are a few other principles at work as well: our growth hormones, and the type of nutrient and exercise that we undertake – but essentially the entire Lean Vegan Work Out will have this formula in mind:

Raise your metabolic rate by raising heartrate (whole body exercises)

+ Eating the right sort of nutrients.

When you start to progress onto the medium and advanced routines, you will find that you might have to work harder to raise your heartrate for that specified time, which in turn *naturally* asks more of your body. This is a good sign, and it means that you are moving your body towards it health potential. You will also start to experience and take advantage of the many good effects of a healthy lifestyle such as a healthy sleeping pattern (which promotes a healthy growth hormone regulation), and higher immune system (allowing you to lose weight quicker, and giving you more general stamina). There will also be a whole number of beneficial other side effects such as better moods, clarity of thought and higher levels of concentration, and a better sex life.

General Health Concerns

Obviously, any practice which is aimed at changing our body has to come with a few caveats, especially if you suffer from any of the following conditions:

- Heart murmurs/heart complaints
- Fragile/brittle bones
- Immuno-system disorders
- Arthritis
- Diabetes
- Or if you are currently pregnant

If you do happen to suffer from any of these, then please take especial care and consult your general health practitioner.

For the rest of us, we will be concentrating on more general health tips, which can be summed up as *Stay Warm, Stay Fuelled,* and *Stay Focussed!*

Stay Warm means that it is important for the muscles and tendons of the body to be in the right state before exercising. This can be done by stretching as well as making sure that you are wearing the correct exercise clothing. Tracksuit bottoms and a short-sleeved shirt should be fine, but also consider yoga pants and special exercise shirts. This will help you to warm up your body and so reduce sprains and strains.

Staying Fuelled means that, whilst you shouldn't exercise on a full stomach, you should also not exercise when starving. Make sure that you are generally eating well in the same weeks that you are exercising.

Staying Focussed is also a vital and important part of avoiding injury – particularly if you are using any sort of free weights. When you are exercising, try to focus upon the actual exercises that you are doing – not on your job or what you might have to do later, or before, etc. Stay in the moment, concentrate upon your surroundings, and the feel of your body. This will provide you with more than enough preparation to avoid most dangers and injuries.

The Work Out Diary

In just the same way as our Vegan Diary, we are going to use a Work Out Diary to track our progress and plan our exercise routine. This will stop us from over-expending our energy, and putting us in the danger zone for tiredness and injuries.

Tip: Injuries predominantly occur at the end of a work-out session, when we are tired and our muscles shaky Be especially careful at this times, and remember to eat well!

In just the same way as our Lean Vegan Meal Diary, we will use a calendar or notebook, and mark down the exercise that we take on what day, including how many repetitions and weights of what sort. In just a few short weeks you will find that you are easily able to up those repetitions and weights, as well as change the exercise plan to accommodate your needs.

It is important to remember that one of the purposes of the Work Out diary is not to castigate or punish oneself for exercising. If we miss a session, we just move onto the next session on the list. It is rather to just motivate, inspire, and keep a track of what we are able to do. You may spend a week doing 30 push-ups every other day, and think to yourself: 'I am going to try 35 next week!' Remember that the goal is aided by you staying positive and having fun!

Another wonderful opportunity offered by the work-out diary is the way that it can mesh with your life. After a month or so, you may be able to collapse your meal diary, diet plan, and work-out diary all into one journal, along with your daily appointments and work schedules. This will help you become more in control of your life, and plan when is the best time to exercise.

Consider these questions when you are working on your Work Out Diary:

- *What days am I the most busy (and have the least amount of time to exercise)?*
- *What days am I usually at my most tired?*
- *What days do I have free time during the morning, afternoon, or evening?*
- *What days/evenings/mornings do I wish to keep to myself as a treat?*

Tip: Remember that it is also very important to rest and recuperate when conducting a healthy exercise regime. You will see from our beginner exercise plans that we have built in some of these 'R-n-R' days, but you may want to swap and change them, as suits your lifestyle.

Mental Strength

You will probably have heard of the phrase 'positive mental attitude', especially in discussions of fitness and exercise. There is nothing that could be more accurate than in saying that it is our expectations that creates our experiences, especially with fitness.

This is why it is also important to consider Mental Strength in any discussion with physical strength. Mental Strength is not the same as 'toughing it out' or 'gritting your teeth' those qualities might well be stamina, endurance, or toughness – but they sound to me as having a lot more in common with stubbornness! A stubborn attitude will get you injured when exercising, whereas even a gentle attitude, when applied with conviction and determination (in other words: mental strength) will get you fit.

As with any health-improvement scheme, you will find that there will be times when you feel too tired to go for that run, or to make that salad, and all you want to do is just eat junk food and watch satellite television. I am not here to moralize or to tell you that you shouldn't – we all need rest days, and we all need to look after yourself.

However, we should also consider mental strength; and by this I mean our determination, our guts, our willingness to have faith in what we are doing – as another spiritual muscle that we are toning. The more we exercise it, the more that we will find that it grows stronger, and the more effective people that we become!

Tip: Consider the question; what does mental strength mean to you?

Step 4

- *Create a Work-Out Diary, choose which plan suits you best (Beginner or Moderate to start with)*
- *Make sure that you have adequate training clothes and equipment (jogging trousers, shirts, or a home weight system).*
- *Consider joining a local gym, or look into local exercise clubs: dancing, walking, running, or swimming.*
- *Choose the first day that you will be starting your Cardio exercise, and mark it in your Work-Out diary. Choose a day that you know you know will have plenty of time to recover afterwards!*

Lean Vegan Exercise Routines

Cardio 1 Exercises

Cardio exercises (short for cardiovascular) work on your circulatory system, primarily your oxygen to blood flow. It gets your heart pumping, and is the surest way to increase your metabolic rate and tone up.

When performing any of these exercises, start slowly, and then progress to the optimum speed which you feel that you can maintain for the time duration. For our Lean Vegan Exercise plan, you should perform 1 Cardio exercise at a time, (only 1 if in the Beginner Routine) per exercise day, or, if you are feeling particularly up to it, you can perform up to 3, but any more would almost certainly tire you out, and risk injury!

- 20 mins Jogging
- 3 sets of 30 Jumping Jacks
- 15 mins Skip-Rope
- 25 mins Swimming
- 25-30 mins Hiking/Strenuous walking
- 30 mins Aerobics class
- 15 mins Cycling

Cardio 2 Exercises

As with Cardio 1 exercises, perform only 1 exercise, particularly if this is also a split day, when you will also either be doing a weights or a core exercise. By varying the types of Cardio that you do, you will help different muscle groups and general body health.

- 30-45 mins Jogging
- 3 X 5 min Sprinting/Running
- 2 X 3 sets of 30 Jumping Jacks
- 2 X 15 mins Skip-Rope
- 35-45 mins Swimming
- 1 Hour Hiking/Strenuous walking
- 1 Hour Aerobics class
- 25 mins Cycling

Weights 1 Exercises

Weights (or sometimes called strength) exercises are many and varied, and you will find that you benefit extensively from joining a local gym. However, with these exercises, as they work on isolated muscle groups, you are quite often able to perform between 3 and five different Weights/Strength exercises every session. Whereas you may only perform 1 Cardio exercise a session, try at least three to four Weights exercises per session.

- 30/20/10 Push-ups
- 15/10/5 Bench Press
- 10/5 Dumbbell Fly-overs
- 15/10/5 Leg Weight Extenders

Weights 2 Exercises

With our Weights 2/Strength exercises, we really want to see the body starting to exert more power. We do this by adding more exercises to our routine (upping the amount from three weights exercises to six per session, say) or by upping the weight used. In body-resistance exercises, such as push-ups, we have our natural body weight to accommodate for this increase in strength, when using free or gym weights however, we will be asking ourselves to increase the weight amount that we practise with by between 5lbs to 10lbs from our weights 1 exercise.

- 40/30/20 Push-ups
- 20/15/10 Bench Press
- 15/10 Dumbbell Fly-overs
- 20/15/10 Leg Weight Extenders

Core 1 Exercises

Core exercises are thought by many as a type of strength exercise, however, due to their slow and balanced nature they work on our endurance rather than our brute strength. Core exercises work on strengthening the body frame as a whole unit, and asks all of our muscles to tighten and tone up. A lot of professional models and lean athletes do a lot of core exercises, as they encourage endurance, stamina, and a lean tone throughout the body. They predominantly use slow positions or movements that we hold for extended amount of time. Yoga is an exceptional example of predominantly Core strength exercises.

When performing Core exercises, always do at least 2 different exercises, with no upper limit to how many you should do per session, other than the necessities of time you have available!

- 30/20/10 Push-ups
- 1 min Plank position (fully arm-extended push up, held and not lowered)
- 1 min Leg Raises (raising each leg at a time, holding in the air, then both legs together, and hold)
- 30/20/10 Sit-Ups
- 20/15/10 Squats
- 25 min Yoga session

Core 2 Exercises

With our Core 2 exercises, we will be performing exactly the same exercises as before, but we may choose to do more exercises per session (for example, push-ups, plank, + leg raises and squats) or we may perform our exercises for longer. You will be surprised at just how demanding and difficult they can be!

- 2 X 30/20/10 Push-ups
- 3 X 1 min Plank position
- 3 X 1 min Leg Raises
- 2 X 30/20/10 Sit-Ups
- 2 X 20/15/10 Squats
- 2 X 25 min Yoga session, or 1 X 45 min Yoga session.

Beginning Routine:

In this routine we will practise building up general stamina, utilizing the beginner light exercises (numbered as '1').

- **Total:** 3 Days on, 4 Days Off (Light)
- Day 1 – Cardio 1
- Day 2 – Rest
- Day 3 – Weights 1
- Day 4 – Rest
- Day 5 – Rest
- Day 6 – Cardio 1 + Core 1
- Day 7 – Rest
- **Duration:** Keep to this routine for at least between 4-6 weeks before moving on to the Moderate/Medium Routine

Medium/Moderate Routine

Designed as the next logical step from the Beginner routine, this exercise plan asks your body to recover at the same rate, with a generous rest-cycle, but also asks it to perform a little more in the way of activity, strength, and tone.

- **Total:** 3 Days on, 4 Days off (Light)
- Day 1 – Cardio 2
- Day 2 – Rest
- Day 3 – Weights 1, Core 1
- Day 4 – Rest
- Day 5 – Rest
- Day 6 – Cardio 1 + Weights 1

- Day 7 – Rest
- **Duration:** Keep to this routine for at least 4 weeks before moving on to the Advanced Routine

Advanced Routine

Designed to increase the amount asked of your body, and really start to build your strength and physical fitness.

- **Total:** 4 Days on, 3 Days off
- Day 1 – Cardio 2
- Day 2 – Rest
- Day 3 –Weights 2, Core 2
- Day 4 – Rest
- Day 5 – Cardio 1
- Day 6 – Core 1 + Weights 2
- Day 7 – Rest
- **Duration:** Try this routine out for a week to start with, and see if your body is over tired or beginning to feel strained. Practice this routine *for no longer* than 3 weeks at a time, before moving back to a Moderate Routine for a week. If, after this changeover you feel healthy and able, advance to Semi-Pro Routines

Semi-Pro Routine

Designed as an optional routine, after you have completed all of the above (4 weeks beginner, 4 weeks of Moderate, 3 week Advanced, 1 week Moderate).

- **Total:** 4 Days on, 3 Days off
- Day 1 – Cardio 2, Weights 1
- Day 2 – Rest
- Day 3 – Cardio 1, Weights 1, Core 1
- Day 4 – Rest
- Day 5 – Weights 2, Core 2
- Day 6 – Rest
- Day 7 – Cardio 1
- **Duration:** Alternate this practice with either the Advanced or Moderate Routines as you need.

Step 5

- *Perform one whole cycle of your chosen routine (4-6 weeks of Beginner) before progressing on to the next stage (4 weeks of Moderate, or 3 weeks of Advanced).*
- *Keep at it until you progress to the next stage (which should take you at least another month).*

Conclusion

Thank you for coming on this journey of health and self-discovery with me! I hope that, by the time that you have reached this far you will be motivated to have already tried out a few of our vegan recipes outlined inside, and brought some running shoes!

This is the first step to a whole new healthier you, and there is yet much more to come on your journey towards health. You may find, after the first couple of months of working with this guide book that your practise deepens and you find many unexpected benefits to the Lean Vegan Diet and Work Out. Perhaps you cycle to work now, and save money on fuel, or have met a lot of new friends through an exercise club or local food market. Maybe you will have even started to grow some of your own tasty vegetables for your own handmade vegan dishes!

Really, the Lean Vegan Diet and Work Out isn't just a diet book or an exercise plan, it is also a lifestyle, one which embraces the healthy, possible future you with open arms. You may well be surprised at how different your life becomes.

Be prepared for greater senses of wellbeing and fitness, as well as sharper thinking, easier sleep and more stable moods. All of these health benefits will impact on your work life, your social life, and any personal relationships that you have. It may sound like a bit of a grand claim, but really it is a very simple one: if you look after yourself, then in turn you will start to look after people around you as well. People respond to that sense of health and vitality, you'll see!

So, the very first steps on your road to the new you would be this: to start documenting what you eat right now (before the diet) and think about how that makes you feel. Start to wonder what you can replace and substitute those meals for. Also start looking at your day-to-day week. Are there any times you can free up for a quick jog, or to go swimming? Remember that this is your future that you are seizing control of, and investing in!

Another wonderful benefit to this approach to life is that it is not exclusive. It is possible to be vegan inside a non-vegan family, and there are plenty of opportunities to encourage others to enjoy the benefits that you are. You do not have to have a gruelling personal exercise regime, when a joint family visit to the swimming pool will also do, as will a large family vegan feast!

In this way I hope that this little book leaves you with a sense of optimism and possibility. Please remember to leave feedback at the marketplace where you brought it, and, if you so wish share your stories and progress of the Lean Vegan Work Out Diet with me there!

Many thanks,

Live Nutritive

p.s. *If you feel you received value from this book we would be forever grateful if you could leave us a review on Amazon*